Tabata Training:

The 4 Minute Workout

By John Paulson

Tabata Training: The 4 Minute Workout

Copyright © 2012 John Paulson

CONTENTS

1. Preface

The Tabata Protocol

In today's world, excuses are abundant. When it comes to hitting the gym regularly, time tops the list of offenders. For this reason, the Tabata workout is the perfect fit (you shall see why later). This material is intended to give you an understanding of the Tabata Protocol Workout, beyond the simplistic " meat" of the activity. After all, who doesn't appreciate dessert and an appetizer with their main course?

We are going to cover the history of the Tabata Workout, the benefits of performing it, goals achievable by incorporating it into your training regimen, the importance of progression and how to put together your very own Tabata Workout.

Interested? You should be. Learn how 4 minutes is enough to take you to the next level.
Now let's get moving!

2. The Tabata Protocol

The Tabata Protocol is an effective, high intensity interval training (HIIT) workout that emphasizes development of both aerobic and anaerobic metabolic pathways. The Tabata Protocol was developed and improved by Dr. Izumi Tabata, a former researcher for The National Institute of Fitness and Sports, in Kanoya, Japan, who first got wind of the workout from a coach of the National Speed Skating Team.

The Tabata Protocol is vastly different, however, from other HIIT cardiovascular workouts, in the sense that it has a profound effect on improving both aerobic and anaerobic exercise capacity, accomplishing this fete in just four minutes. The method to achieve these results in not hard to grasp, but it will be hard to handle, at least in the beginning, since exceeding 100% of your VO2 (maximum oxygen uptake), will leave you feeling like a train just hit you.

Tabata Intervals

Tabata intervals refer to the time under which you are performing exercise against the time you are at rest. In a typical Tabata Workout session, intervals follow the pattern of 20 seconds of work, followed by 10 seconds of rest (or low intensity work) and repeated for a total of 4 minutes (or 8 intervals). The aim of these work intervals is to perform as much work as humanly possible (at the highest intensity) to surpass the fatigue threshold and develop improved cardiovascular function (among many other benefits).

It is important to note that while maximum work exertion is relative to each person, the original research conducted by Dr. Tabata found it necessary to perform the exercise at 170% VO2. Achieving 100% is difficult for most people, so while not set in stone, the aim is to work as hard as your body can handle in that period of time.

Repetitions

Tabata Training originally was catered towards Tri-athletes, who required a high level of muscular endurance. As such, much of the original research was conducted on a stationery cycle, recording duration of work, not repetitions.

However, new Tabata workouts including resistance training involve performing the maximum number of *repetitions*, not intensity per se. The number of repetitions performed in such a workout is not of great importance, but what *is important* is that you do record the number of reps you do manage, as a benchmark for improvement.

A practice referred to as Tabata Scoring is very useful here; you just make a visual note of the minimum number of repetitions performed during the workout, and use that as an indicator to surpass it in the next workout. For example, if you managed 8 reps in the last interval, strive for 9 next time.

3. Benefits of Tabata Workouts

The benefits gained from performing Tabata workouts are enormous and improve quality of life significantly. Benefits derived from performing Tabata Workouts may include:

Improving Cardiovascular Health

Due of involvement of both aerobic and anaerobic metabolic pathways, Tabata protocol workouts elicit a very favorable effect on cardiovascular health. The aerobic component of the exercise improves the amount of oxygen the muscles are able to utilize during a period of time, in this case, exercise. Improving aerobic capacity has numerous effects on functional capacity of the body such as:

Improving strength of the muscles involved in respiration, such as the diaphragm, lungs and a range of accessory muscles. This effectively helps to make the passage of air in and out of the lungs easier.

Improving circulation- the muscles in the heart are strengthened and are subject to mild hypertrophy (growth), which improves the ability of it to pump blood. As a result, blood pressure is favorably reduced, the heart rate at rest is decreased (pulse), and the rate of recovery is improved significantly since nutrients reach the sites of muscle breakdown quickly.

Improved Recovery

Tabata Protocol based workouts will over time, improve the time it takes you to recover between intervals, and day to day. Initially, you will be sore; possibly for days after, however, after the first six weeks or so, you will notice a significant improvement in the time it takes for you to recover following a session. In addition, persons who weight train are likely to feel less post-workout pain and be able to perform more repetitions for a given exercise.

Enhanced Conditioning

Conditioning is not universal across all sports disciplines; rather it means different thing to different athletes. For endurance athletes(such as tri-athletes) conditioning enables the heart to supply blood in a more efficient manner, allowing exchange of carbon dioxide and oxygen, and helping to remove mild accumulation of lactic acid.

For strength training athletes, or those involved in intense short-burst activity, incorporating Tabata workouts will enable longer anaerobic training capacity, as well as help with harnessing explosive ability and will not sabotage strength and muscle gains, as most low to moderate intensity cardiovascular activities are notorious in doing.

Excellent Progression Tracking

Tabata training offers a method to objectively track progression over a period of time. Although Tabata training can be continued indefinitely, cycles normally run for between 6- 8 weeks, to ensure the nervous system does not become over trained, as is common in many high intensity training protocols.

For a first timer, it may be a good idea to start with less than the standard 8 intervals, since the original study conducted by Dr. Izumi Tabata involved extremely fit individuals. Tracking involves recording the number of reps performed during each interval, the lowest rep interval attained, and sometimes the average number of reps per interval (these all apply to resistance-bases Tabatas). Tabatas performed with cardiovascular equipment need to focus on tension and other variables instead of repetitions.

4. Improvements Gained Through Tabata Workouts

Strength

Thanks to the anaerobic component of Tabata training, short duration intense training benefits significantly. It is a great add on for strength athletes and bodybuilders to employ, since catabolism (muscle breakdown) will not be a side effect of training, and strength will not be inhibited through the cortisol loop.

Recovery Time

The improved state of the cardiovascular system, achieved via Tabata workouts, will allow blood to flow faster to sites that need nutrients for repair to begin. The result is a more potent anabolic response, and faster recovery since waste materials will be, in like manner, eliminated rapidly.

Nervous System

While the original test subjects under Dr. Tabata performed the workouts 4 days a week, in addition to another day of moderate intensity activity, this is not the best approach for achieving the full effect of the workout. Such intensity would wreak havoc on the nervous system, leading to an overtraining syndrome and restriction of explosive gains(strength, speed etc.) incorporating the workout once or twice per week is plenty for improving firing of nervous system synapses and improving the neuromuscular conductivity.

Mental Endurance

Nothing can prepare you for the willpower this workout will require; it is not for the faint of heart. You may initially fail to achieve all 8 intervals in the stipulated 4 minute limit, however, you will build unbreakable mental prowess after just a few weeks of performing Tabata workouts.

Physical Endurance

Tabata workouts are great for increasing physical endurance, measured by the ability of an athlete to maintain aerobic capacity over increasing time periods. Moderate intensity cardiovascular activity performed for an hour 5 times weekly for 6 weeks has been shown to improve aerobic capacity by a decent 7%.

Tabata workouts, done for 4 minutes, 4 times weekly for 6 weeks was demonstrated to improve aerobic capacity by a massive 14%, and anaerobic capacity by over 25%! Incorporating these workouts will take you to the outer limits of your endurance threshold.

Flexibility

Tabatas improve flexibility through a type of muscle fiber stretching known as ballistic stretching. This type of stretching involves rapid movements through a muscle ROM (range of motion) leading to an adaptation of the joint to accommodate the exercise easier.

Balance

Tabata workouts are to a large degree lower body based; as a result, a significant improvement to balance, and subsequently posture is commonly observed. The quadriceps (front-thigh muscle) along with the posterior chain (hips, glutes, and hamstrings) is frequently recruited during the movements in a Tabata workout, strengthening the base of the body.

5. Goals of Tabata Workouts

Improving Reflexes

Tabata workouts can significantly improve one aspect of reflex training; reaction time. As if accurate timing of the intervals is not enough to get your response time into third gear, the development of the lower body muscles will also facilitate this feat. Explosive movements, such as plyometric training incorporated into a Tabata workout will improve reflexes even more.

Strengthening the Nervous System

Tabata workouts performed just a few times weekly will improve nervous system compensation in response to exercise. However, performing numerous times weekly might not be the best idea as overtraining is likely to occur (from a CNS burnout).

Improving Emotional Well Being

Neurotransmitters and hormones play a large role in determining emotions and moods, a goal that will be improved with Tabata training. By strengthening the nervous system, and the synapses that bridge nerves, neurotransmitters and hormones are better able to mediate their effects, and counter abnormalities, such as may occur in depression (caused by a serotonin synaptic anomaly).

Improving Physical Well Being

The ease of the heart to pump oxygenated blood throughout the body is one of the effects that facilitate all round physical well being. By also promoting anaerobic capacity, more intense short duration activities can be handles with relative ease.

Improving Stamina

As you progress in a Tabata workout, it is likely that 4 minutes will not seem enough. In such cases, more "sets" may be added to your progression. More sets refer to performing more 4 minute workouts, since conditioning is continually being achieved. Eventually, the duration of a single set may be prolonged to make the workout even more challenging.

Measurable Goals to Improve On

The number of reps- as you progress in a Tabata workout, your lowest achieved rep range will be surpassed.

So if you achieve 10 reps today, you have a clearly defined goal to surpass the next time.

Rep intensity- the rep intensity can be increased by adding weight when possible and increasing the number of reps performed.

The Number of Intervals per Workout- a typical workout will have 8 intervals, however as you progress you may be able to either increase the number of intervals, thus exceeding the 4 minute zone, or add on more 4 minute segments, effectively performing more sets.

Performing Tabatas

The most common Tabata workout protocol is performed in the ratio of 2:1 (work: rest) and translates to 20 seconds: 10 seconds. The most common variations to the workout are

20:10 intervals

This is the most common interval timing, and is the best option for first timers. To begin with, 8 intervals are assigned to be completed during a 4 minute period, which may be extended as stamina develops.

60:30 intervals

While still being equal to the 2:1 ratio, which is the popular protocol, this variation is used mainly in highly conditioned athletes who have successfully completed the 20:10 workout. The downside to this method is that intensity suffers, since it is difficult to maintain VO2 of over 100% for periods exceeding 20 seconds.

180:60

This is the most brutal variation of the Tabata workout, and is only undertaken by a handful of elite athletes. Like the 60:30 method, intensity falters greatly during this period, questioning the rationale of employing it in the first place. It may take some years for a novice athlete to ever achieve the level of conditioning required for this variation.

The Standard Tabata

This is the best method for most athletes, each interval taking a total of 30 seconds (20 work and 10 rest). Many variations have been tested, including alternating differing exercises during 20 second work periods, and while it does help to keep good form in check, there is simply not enough rest periods in between to change exercises, or the need to maintain perfect form.

In more conditioned athletes, multiple 4 minute Tabatas may be performed. The time between these Tabatas should be 1 minute, to allow some clearance of lactic acid from the body.

6. The Importance of Progression in Tabata Workouts

The basis of receiving maximum benefit from any workout is progression. The body is a marvelous machine, one that tries as much as possible to stay just the way it is.

However, it is also very willing to adapt to changes, if the stimulus is there and it sees the need to. You will never come anywhere near your fitness goals if day after day, month after month, you keep doing the same thing, without ever increasing the intensity (the reps performed, weight used etc.). Progression is necessary if you want to:

Prevent plateaus

A plateau is the point reached where your body simply cannot continue to progress, due to numerous factors, such as overtraining, not getting enough sleep or skimpy nutrition. Most persons will eventually hit a plateau regardless of their choice of exercise, the reason being simple; you cannot push the body beyond human limits.

Do not expect to be able to squat 2000 pounds even though you are progressing at 50 pounds per week, it is impossible. Tabata workouts allow the body to handle short burst exercise up to 25% better (anaerobic ability), and maintain moderate intensity for 15% longer. This translates to delayed plateauing.

Improve the Nervous System

High intensity exercise, such as Tabata workouts, primes the nervous system to strengthen neuromuscular junctions, to facilitate stronger muscle contractions. It is important to keep in mind that more is not better when using Tabata workouts, so keep it short and infrequent.

Make Exercises More Challenging

It should be obvious that performing sprints at 20mph will be tougher than a casual 5mph; such is the tenet of the Tabata Protocol. For short periods, you will keep increasing the intensity, until the need arises to increase the number of intervals. The number of repetitions performed as well as the weight used may all help to make the exercise more challenging.

Tabata Workouts are Easy to Track

For most of the workout, the time remains fixed, while the repetitions and weight used may increase from time to time. The focus off of the total time can allow you to focus on more important figures such as the repetition count and eventually the increasing number of intervals.

Methods to Add Progression

Increase the number of repetitions performed during any given interval- being able to perform more repetitions with the same weight represents an adaptation to training and progress.

Increase the number of intervals per workout-advanced athletes who find that a simple 4 minute workout no longer gives them results may add on additional intervals. Although the repetitions and weights should preferentially be increased over extending the work time, when a plateau with either occurs increasing the intervals is an effective solution.

Increase the difficulty of exercise- for example, if using a stationery cycle, increase the tension when you are completing all 8 intervals with relative ease. If performing weight bearing exercise, slight variations to the movement may increase the difficulty(such as changing stance)

Increase weight used- this is the most effective and common progression technique; it will provide years of work without reaching the limiting plateau.

Note: Do not attempt to add in more progression until you are capable of performing the Tabata intervals easily and correctly.

7. Putting Together Your Tabata Workout

Once you've understood the appetizers, it's time to progress to the meat of it all; the actual workout. Though many persons jump straight into the workout without necessary preparatory work, we strongly advise against it since cold muscles are likely to cause injuries easily. Warm ups are great at increasing blood flow prior to the workout and priming the body for work. A good approach follows this structure:

Warm Up

A warm up period of 10- 15 minutes at about 50% VO2 max is enough to get the blood pumping and get joints supple and ready for activity. Do not increase the intensity during a warm up as you are likely to be fried by the time the real workout comes around.

Joint Mobility Drills

These are done to decrease the occurrence of injuries, and to encourage your joints to move through a full range of motion. Stiff joints or lack of joint mobility is a large contributing factor to injuries while exercising, by simply performing one joint specific mobility drill daily, you can significantly decrease the risk of developing an injury.

Circulation Moves

Performing dynamic stretching improves blood flow by mimicking the motion of exercise. It induces cellular and metabolic pathways, some of which signal cAMP (cyclical adenosine monophosphate), a potent natural vasodilator.

The Tabata

As you should be familiar with by now, you will perform each Tabata interval for 30 seconds, composed of 20 seconds work, and 10 seconds rest (either at a stop or low intensity). This cycle is repeated 8 times for a total of 4 minutes. The actual activity performed can vary, and consist either of cardiovascular work or weighted exercise. As you progress, it is a good idea to perform multiple Tabata sets, each consisting of the same 4 minutes total time. It is important to take a structured minute or rest in between each set, and you can work up to a total 5 work sets.

Cool Downs

The term cool down refers to slowly bringing down your heart rate, instead of just coming to a dead stop. By cooling down, you decrease the risk of fainting due to pooling of blood in the work muscles, remove lactic acid which is shown to clear best under slow- moderate exercise. Finally, the greatest benefit of a cool down is to help prepare your body for the upcoming workout, normally in a few days.

Flexibility, Mobility and Stretching

The joint mobility drills are done again, with the intention of relaxing tense muscles. Static stretching is also done at this time, which has been shown to greatly decrease the occurrence of DOMS (delayed onset muscle soreness), and to return the work muscles to their relaxed state. Releasing this constriction of blood around the muscle also allows waste materials to be cleared faster and nutrient delivery to begin.

Choice of Exercises

When selecting an exercise, it is important to choose one that does not require too much assembly, or downtime while preparing for the next interval. One of the most common exercises is sprinting and walking, which requires no preparation; just do it!

Lower Body

Jump rope, step ups, lunges (bodyweight or with added weight), sprinting and walking, and the front squat.

Upper Body

Pushups, pull ups, inverted rows, and barbell cleans are good options for the upper body.

Core

Crunches/ Sit ups, leg raises and V ups (simultaneously raising the shoulders and the legs straight up to touch (in a v shape).

As we advocated earlier, it is generally not a good idea to perform multiple exercises within a single 4 minute period. However, if performing multiple sets, there is no problem performing exercises for different body parts.

8. Closing Words

The most important tool to have when performing Tabata workouts is an effective stop watch, preferably one that is programmable for the 4 minutes with a beep signaling the end of each interval. Additionally, if you prefer to work out at home, a good stationery cycle with a timer, treadmill, or barbell or dumbbell set will be more than enough to get the burn of your life.

Performing Tabata will get you in the best shape of your life-Period. However, it is not easy to accomplish, and you should get the clear from your Physician before embarking on the Protocol. It is intended for normal- healthy individuals to improve their fitness level.